TEA CLEANSE

CHALLENGE

7 Day Tea Cleanse Reset To Lose 10 Pounds And Get That Flat Belly You've Always Wanted

Table of Contents

Introduction

I want to thank you and congratulate you for downloading the book, "Tea Cleanse Challenge: 7 Day Tea Cleanse Reset to Lose 10 Pounds and Get That Flat Belly You've Always Wanted".

This book contains proven steps and strategies on how to shed the extra pounds and live a healthier, happier lifestyle.

Why is it that when most people think of health and fitness, their first instinct is to feel discouraged and act as though the whole idea doesn't exist? Sure we can't all be fitness experts, but if you're really serious about getting back into shape, there are techniques that can help you work for that body you've always wanted. Whether it's losing weight or having more energy, going on a tea cleanse is one of the most effective ways to get started on a healthier lifestyle.

While your body's natural capacity to burn stored fat can slow down with age, that doesn't mean that you should give up on your fitness goals. No matter what stage of life you're in, there's still so much you can do to improve your physical, mental, and physical wellbeing and reading this book is the first step to living the life you've always wanted.

This book is designed to teach you how to start living a healthier greener lifestyle by going on a tea cleanse. This isn't meant to be a fad diet to help you lose weight fast, but it should encourage you to use tea detox to make healthier lifestyle choices, and reset your lifestyle in the process.

Who is this Book For?

- For people who are sick and tired of going on crash diets that just don't work.

- For people who want to use their energy to build strength.

- For people who want to make healthier food choices and get back to a normal eating routine.

- ....and many more!

So what are you waiting for? Start reading and make that change in your lifestyle today!

Thanks again for downloading this book, I hope you enjoy it!

Don't forget to check out one of my favourite diets at the bottom:

Chapter 1 - How Detox Tea can Help You

Detoxification gained a nasty reputation these past years. While there are countless detox products that claim to be "the only weight loss solution", we all know by now that liquid diets simply don't work on their own. You may experience a sudden drop in your weight in the beginning, but usually that also means a drop in nutrients and energy. It may help you jumpstart your weight loss journey, but it also gets difficult to sustain along the way.

A tea detox, or teatox as most celebrities like to call it, is a much healthier approach to detoxifying your body. Instead of replacing full meals with a liquid drink, you only need to add a few cups of herbal tea to your already existing, nourishing diet. This means that you can still have all the fruits and vegetables you want even while you're trying to cleanse your body of all the harmful toxins that are trapped in your bloodstream.

Because detox tea is so easy to incorporate into anyone's lifestyle, it's no wonder that countless celebrities now swear by its amazing effects. What is it about tea that makes it the best weight loss solution on the market today? Here's how tea can help you get started on a healthier and happier way of life.

According to a 2013 study conducted by American researches, going on a tea drinking binge has a wide array of benefits that covers almost every area of the human body. From lowering your risk of stroke, to increasing mental performance, tea is packed with catechins that can help elevate your energy level even with less calorie consumption. This is probably the main reason why tea drinkers cope better both physically and emotionally when they make changes on their lifestyle.

High quality teas, both green and black, are rich in antioxidants that can help boost the body's natural cleansing ability. Antioxidants play a crucial role in the detoxification process because it reduces oxidative stress levels significantly and gets rid of free radicals from the body. While drinking tea alone isn't enough to get the job done, it can still make the process much easier for the body. It's considered as harmless in comparison to many detox products designed to just mess up the body's natural cycle.

Because there are teas specifically blended with additional ingredients like lemongrass, dandelion, and even milk thistle, you're sure to get more benefits from doing a teatox than a traditional detox. You can choose the perfect tea blend that will help you meet your specific health and fitness goals. If you're looking for a detoxifying drink that will alleviate stress on the liver, an herbal infusion with ginger for example, can clean your bloodstream more efficiently. It's just a matter of finding the right tea blend that will suit not just your mood or taste, but also complement your body system.

However, keep in mind that not all teatox teas are created equally. Some contain a very powerful detoxifying but dangerous ingredient called senna. Senna is an herbal laxative that stimulates the intestines to purge its contents. While this ingredient can be helpful on the body for a short amount of time, taking too much senna for too long can have devastating effects on the digestive system. It can cause electrolyte balance which if you're not careful, can lead to dehydration. If you feel constipated, taking senna tea for a few nights can be helpful but don't let it become your everyday cup.

So when's the best time to take your cup of tea? Health experts believe that you can take it whenever you feel like it, as long as you make the effort to drink more water throughout the day since most tea blends contain caffeine. However, for tea drinkers who can only stomach 1-2 cups of tea per day, it's best to take their first cup upon waking up, and the second one before preparing for bed. This way, they will get their dose of antioxidants without having to make any major changes in their daily routine.

Whatever teatox blend you choose, make sure that you eat a healthy diet with it. Going on a tea detox can only do so much without the help of a proper diet plan. If you want to detoxify your body, you need to make that life changing decision to cut out processed foods from your food plan. You need to feed your body with fruits, vegetables, and whole grains in order to enhance your digestive system's natural cycle. Once you start getting the hang of eating clean, detoxifying your system is going to be a breeze.

Chapter 2 - Green Tea Facts

Green tea has become all the rage these past years. Ever since medical studies have come out of their apparent weight loss effects, people from all over the world have been choosing green tea over the usual brew. However, while you may feel like you're getting healthier with every sip of green tea, you need to get the facts straight in order to take full advantage of the benefits. What is it exactly about this drink that is making people go crazy for it? Here are a few green tea facts that you definitely need to know.

Green tea can boost a sluggish metabolism

Even as our metabolism slows down as we age, genetics also affects how our bodies use up calories and stored fat. If you're one of those who can't seem to burn fat as fast as you should, then including green tea into your daily diet may just be the perfect solution for you. Countless studies have proven that green tea can enhance your body's natural ability to burn up fat. Of course, you'll need to lessen your sugar intake and increase your vegetable consumption for maximum effect, but a cup of green tea every morning should be enough to fire up a sluggish metabolism.

Green tea can lower bad cholesterol levels

Another amazing fact about green tea is that it can significantly lower cholesterol levels, particularly LDL or what we call bad cholesterol. Research shows that people who consume 4 cups of green tea or more daily are less likely to develop high LDL levels that have been linked to many forms of heart disease. If 4 cups seem like too much for you, then you can always opt to take green tea pills that are available in many health stores.

Green tea can stop some cancer in its tracks

Studies also prove that drinking freshly brewed green tea regularly can help reduce your risk of certain cancer that affects the prostate, ovarian, endometrial, and breast. Even on people who have already been diagnosed, drinking green tea can have a positive effect. Why? Because it contains exorbitant amounts of antioxidants that fight off free radicals. The more antioxidants you have in your body, the better your body will be able to cope with elements that attack it from within.

Green tea can lower your diabetes risk

While there still isn't much study on the effects of green tea on a person's sugar levels, drinking at least 2 cups each day can help reduce appetite and curb sugar cravings. In effect, drinking green tea can help you lessen your carbohydrate and sugar intake, which can then lower your risk of developing type 2 diabetes.

Green tea can enhance overall brain functions

Green tea doesn't just have a calming effect, but also a positive effect on brain functions. New research shows that drinking green tea is an easy way to enhance short-term recall and improve memory functions. Although further testing is recommended on the effects green tea can have on other brain functions, it shows great promise in possibly helping combat memory related diseases like Alzheimer's.

As you see, using green tea as your main tea detox agent has many other benefits other than keeping your waistline down. Try drinking an average of 3-10 cups each day if you want to reap the benefits. Again, you don't have to totally deprive yourself of food once you go on a tea detox. As long as you eat clean, you'll be able to see a drastic change in your weight, and your way of life in no time.

Chapter 3 - The One Day Cleanse

What many dieters fail to realize is that the word cleanse is really a verb, and not a noun. If you're not going to make that conscious decision to live a much healthier lifestyle, then all the effort is bound to go to waste. You should look at this detox as a means to help you reach a long-term goal, and not just a short-term fix. Even though this process is called the one day cleanse, it's designed to help you jumpstart what hopefully turns out to be a long-term journey. It's about making the right decisions in order to change all areas of your current lifestyle.

If you're new to the cleansing program, you first need to take a step back and really understand your motives for doing this. Are you doing a cleanse to fit into that wedding dress or are you getting into the program in order to be healthier? While there are technically no wrong or right motives for wanting to do a tea cleanse, there are however motives that will determine how you are able to handle it. You need to build your motives around long-term goals if you want to succeed in this journey.

You also need to be patient towards the entire process, especially if you want to avoid any drastic side effects that could happen when you recklessly rush through the tea cleanse. If you get on with it too fast, your body will overwork your organs and there's a chance that they will only give in. A hasty approach will lead you to bouts of nausea, breakouts, and even headaches so it's always best to allow your body to go through its natural course.

Short-term programs will only push the toxicity around and not properly get rid of it. The key is to allow your body to work at its own pace and follow a plan that will help you reach your long-term weight loss goals, even if that means you'll need to develop a strong sense of discipline along the way.

So how do we do this one day cleanse anyway? Since detoxifying is one of the most effective ways to get our bodies and minds back into top shape, it's important that we find the perfect balance between physical and mental well being. Remember that this one day is primarily designed to help you develop long term habits. It's sad that other cleanses only put importance on what numbers you should see on the scale after your cleanse, and not on how you should feel once you're done. This is why, aside from preparing physically, you should also prepare mentally.

So let's get started, shall we?

The first step is to stock up on fresh lemon juice. The lemon is considered as nature's medicine and is capable of healing and mending cells in your body. No wonder that when it comes to just about any cleanse, lemon plays a huge role in ensuring that the body still functions properly even with the external stress.

Boost your liver's detoxifying function by having a warm glass of lemon water first thing in the morning of your tea detox. Instead of waking your system up with a cup of Joe, drink lemon water to give a zap of energy, minus the dehydration. Squeeze half a lemon into a mug of warm water and turn this drink into your daily morning habit. Need a hint of sweetness? You can always add honey according to taste.

Next, prepare yourself a green smoothie that will give you all the vitamins and minerals your body will need to last through the day. Simply blitz ½ head of spinach, ½ head of romaine lettuce, 3 celery sticks, 1 pear, 1 banana, and 1 apple with 2 large glasses of water. Squeeze ½ of a lemon into the smoothie and mix well before drinking. Drinking this green smoothie to replace all your major meals throughout the day will not only cleanse your system, but also provide your body with the fiber and enzymes it needs to push the toxins out Just because you're on a detox doesn't mean that you should deprive yourself of nature's goodness.

Replace your morning snack with a detox tea that will help you combat midday cravings and leave you feeling refreshed. To prepare the detox tea, simply steep a ginger tea teabag in a cup of freshly boiled water for 2-3 minutes, depending on how strong you want the ginger flavor to come through. Add a squeeze of lemon and a dash of cayenne powder before drinking. These 3 ingredients work together in breaking up the toxins in your body, and at the same time shielding your internal organs from any infections. It may be an acquired taste for some, but that can always be fixed with a quick drizzle of organic honey.

Feeling famished by dinner time? Then it's time to prepare yourself a meal consisting of dark leafy greens and sliced vegetables. Dark leafy vegetables, together with some crunchy vegetables will give your body loads of fiber for the night ahead. You can even spice it up with some cayenne powder if you want to fire up your digestive system and get it burning more calories. While you're doing a cleanse, it would be best to stick to raw and organic vegetables so that you don't put too much pressure on your stomach when it's time to digest. Keep your dinner light.

Eating meat will only derail you from your goals so at this point, it's best to avoid all temptations. Since it's only going to be for one day, you can do away with food items that contain any form of preservatives as well. You may also want to avoid tomatoes (because of its acidity) and avocados (because of its high fat content) on this day since these 2 food items can set you back from your total cleanse. If you want to have a speedy cleanse, you'll need to do a bit more research to see which seemingly harmless fruits and vegetables you'll need to avoid.

You've made it this far so don't commit the most common faux pas when going on a cleanse – eating anything with even the slightest hint of unhealthy fat. Look for cholesterol free alternatives like coconut oil. This source of medium chain fatty acid is packed with benefits such as protecting your body from bacterial attacks and supporting your thyroid's functions. However, for a successful cleanse, do make the effort to limit your oil intake, at least while you're doing this one day cleanse.

The one day cleanse isn't an overnight fix so don't expect to lose more than a couple of pounds once you're through. It's just a step in the right direction as you incorporate more tea detox drinks into your diet and put an end to your unhealthy eating choices. Make sure to ease yourself into this cleanse the best way you can and start taking responsibility over your decisions. After all, you know just how far you need to go. Follow these guidelines and you'll start to see the best version of yourself unfold in just a few short weeks.

Chapter 4 - Tea Detox Recipes to Try Today

Tea detox drinks may seem exciting in the beginning but it can also get monotonous if you'll be drinking the same tea drink every day. Just because you want to lose weight badly doesn't mean that you should settle for the same tea drink every single day. If you want to explore the different tea detox drinks that can supply your body with all the antioxidants it needs while boosting your overall wellbeing, then here are some tea recipes that you need to try today.

Green Tea Smoothie

What do you get when you mix green tea with kale and apple in one smoothie? A drink that is packed with antioxidants and phytonutrients. This smoothie isn't just tasty, but it also keeps your body in top shape in terms of daily nutrition. The yogurt provides a smooth and interesting taste to this fruit and veggie combo. Just one drink and you'll be feeling amazing for hours.

Fun and tasty ingredients:

- 1 cup of brewed green tea, chilled

- ½ red apple

- 1/3 cup baby kale

- 1 tablespoon Greek yogurt

- ½ tablespoon organic honey

- Ice (optional)

How to:

Blend all the ingredients together until you get a think smoothie consistency. If you want a creamy finish without the yogurt, you can try substituting with ½ cup of fresh avocado instead. This won't just give you added fiber, but it will also give you the potassium your body needs while on a tea detox.

Energy Boost Tea Shake

Green tea is famous for being the other source of caffeine so if you need a quick perk me up in the morning, this is the perfect drink while you're on a tea detox. Having half the caffeine content of a regular cup of coffee, this energy boost shake is enough to wake you up, without going into a caffeine shock. Plus, the orange and banana combo is a great way to start off your mornings.

Fun and tasty ingredients:

- 1 teaspoon green tea matcha powder

- 1 cup coconut milk

- ½ orange, deseeded

- 1 medium banana

- ½ tablespoon organic honey

- Ice (optional)

How to:

Blend all the ingredients until you get the consistency of a thick shake. If you feel it lacks body, you can add ½ of a banana into the mix. You can also add a tablespoon of protein powder if you want this drink to replace your first meal of the day. When taken daily, this shake should leave you feeling full and satisfied until lunch time.

Tropical Detox Smoothie

Tropical fruits such as papaya and mango can really add to the flavor profile of this smoothie. Not only do they pack in some serious nutrients, their colors also make the drink very nice to look at. Aside from the antioxidants, ginger tea is a potent drink that will help boost your immunity against infections and diseases. Give this smoothie a whirl if you're looking for an exciting way to get your detox on.

Fun and tasty ingredients:

- 1 cup of brewed ginger tea, chilled

- 1 cup coconut milk

- ½ cup papaya, cubed

- ½ cup mango, cubed

- 1 medium banana

- Ice (optional)

How to:

Blend all the ingredients until you get just the right creamy consistency. Feel free to change up the fruits depending on what's in season. Always choose fresh fruit every chance you get if you want to enjoy maximum nutrition.

Fruity Berry Tea Detox Smoothie

Are you looking for a fresh and healthy alternative to your pre-workout energy drink? Whip up this dandelion and green tea smoothie and you're all set for your workout. The berries will give your body real energy to sustain you through whatever activity you enjoy doing. Make this your tasty daily exercise drink and you'll always look forward to working out.

Fun and tasty ingredients:

- 1 cup of brewed dandelion tea, chilled

- ½ teaspoon green tea matcha powder

- ¼ cup raspberries

- ¼ cup raspberries

- 1 tablespoon Greek yogurt

- Ice (optional)

How to:

Blend all the ingredients until you get a thick creamy consistency. If you're conscious about the calorie count of green yogurt, you can always use a low fat substitute. Add a teaspoon of honey if this recipe is too tart for your taste.

Ginger Tea Spiced Tonic

Who thought that mixing up ginger tea with some spices will result to a health tonic that will help you lose weight and enhance your immune system? This drink isn't just great after a big meal, but it also works wonders when flu season comes around. The only way to get your body back on track when it's being attacked is by flooding it with all the nutrients that it can handle. Doctor's orders!

Fun and tasty ingredients:

- 3 ginger tea teabags

- ¼ teaspoon organic cinnamon

- ¼ teaspoon turmeric

- 8 ounces near boiling purified water

- 1 tablespoon organic honey

How to:

Steep the tea bags in a tea pot and add the spices and honey. Once the tea is ready, remove the tea bags and enjoy. Try experimenting with different spices if you're looking for an exotic brew. For a refreshing aftertaste, squeeze half a lemon into the pot before serving.

Green Frappe

Want to indulge yourself with a drink that will make you feel like you're sipping at your leisure in a high end coffee shop? Then whip up this green frappe and get your daily dose of rich green tea flavor, without the tedious process of brewing tea bags and waiting for your drink to cool down. The matcha powder is packed with the same health benefits, minus the prep time.

Fun and tasty ingredients:

- 1 teaspoon green tea matcha powder

- ½ tablespoon organic honey

- 1 cup coconut milk

- Ice (optional)

Blend all the ingredients until you get a creamy frothy drink. Since you'll only be using a few key ingredients, you can enjoy the richness of this drink at just about any time that you please. The green frappe is best enjoyed alone in the hot summer months or with friends as you talk about your amazing weight loss journey so far.

Awesome Start Tea Juice

Green tea gets a fruity punch from 3 highly nutritious fruits. The pineapple adds fiber while the pear lends the sweetness, and the papaya? Well it gives this drink a unique flavor profile while adding loads of vitamin C. Whip up this drink when you're feeling weak or feverish and you'll be back on your feet in no time. Talk about getting maximum protection from damage caused by free radicals.

Fun and tasty ingredients:

- 1 cup of brewed green tea, chilled

- ½ cup pineapple chunks

- ½ cup pear, cubed

- ½ cup papaya, cubed

How to:

Blend all the ingredients until you get a juice. Make sure to blend until all chunks of fruit have been liquidized. It may take a while to reach that consistency so if you're pressed for time, you can use a strainer to take away the chunky bits before you enjoy your drink.

Chapter 5 - The 7 Day Flat Tummy Weight Loss Plan

Is it really possible to get a flatter tummy in just 7 days? While it may seem impossible to sustain a tea detox for the long term, getting your act together in 7 days can have a huge effect on your body. Try not to think of these 7 days as a quick fix to a problem, but rather as a transition stage that will help you make better food choices and healthier lifestyle decisions. You can talk about detoxifying all you want but the truth is, without a concrete plan, you won't get the results that you want.

This is why this plan is designed to make that transition towards a healthier you much more bearable. It's about introducing gradual changes so that your body doesn't fall into shock. All you need to do is follow this plan to the tee and you'll be seeing a new you in 7 short days.

Monday

The best way to start off your detox is by getting into the habit of drinking more water. The body often confuses thirst with hunger so if you always feel hungry, then that's your body saying you're not drinking enough water. Staying hydrated is a key element in detoxifying and it's also a safe and effective way to boost your energy, especially when you're minimizing your calorie intake. Drink one glass of water before mealtime and another glass right after. This way you'll feel satisfied even without additional food intake.

Tuesday

Once you're body is properly hydrated, the next step is to start the tea detox. Doing the 1 day cleanse that you've read in the earlier chapter should be much easier to do on the second day since you've in effect, minimized your food intake with all the water you drank. This is also the perfect time to stop yourself from indulging on liquid calories. Tuesday is the day you rethink your drink choices in everyday life. Soft drinks, fruit juices, and alcohol are loaded with sugar that you wouldn't want in your system anyway so make it your personal goal to quit the habit on this day.

Wednesday

Make mealtime an occasion even if you'll only be eating fruits and vegetables on this day. Your body may not be well equipped to handle digesting protein and fats after doing the 1 day fast so try not to get too excited. Stick to steamed and lightly seasoned vegetables to get your fill for the day. Fruits are great if you find yourself craving for something sweet. Don't let the tea detox leave you feeling deprived, instead get excited about eating right. And no matter how busy you get, it's important that you set aside time when you can just sit back, relax, and enjoy your meal. When you keep on rushing your meals, you're more likely to overeat because you don't take the time to actually chew your food and allow the body to feel full on its own.

Thursday

Do you have a snacking habit? Then dedicate this day to get rid of that "treat" mentality. Just because you feel stressed or you worked out a bit, it does not give you an excuse to indulge on all your favorite treats like chocolates and chips. These treats are often loaded with calories and fat so rewarding yourself with all the tasty treats you can think of only validates the idea in your head that it's okay to eat them. Look for healthier alternatives like fruits and nuts if you want to satisfy your sweet and salty cravings.

Friday

Friday is about developing new habits to correspond your healthier lifestyle. This includes correcting your sleeping habits and getting into your exercise groove. Studies show that people who don't get enough sleep are more likely to overeat so if you want to stop the cravings, you need to increase your snooze time. Try going to bed at a set time and avoid playing with your gadgets during bedtime. That should be enough to set the mood for some quality sleep. While not everyone gets excited by the idea of exercising, you need to find a way to psyche yourself for it. Start by taking a morning or night walk, or if you're feeling adventurous, you can try doing a 10 minute HIIT beginner exercise sequence. The point is to start somewhere and turn it into a daily habit.

Saturday

If you've followed the schedule, by now you should be feeling a bit healthier and a little less famished. Celebrate the weekend by eating well balanced meals. Your meals should contain healthy servings of carbs, protein, and healthy fats. Settle for any less and you're bound to feel hungry in a couple of hours. Satisfy your craving for meat and fat by having a healthy serving of white fish in a light olive oil sauce.

Sundays

Get into the habit of planning your meals from this day on so that you have all your nutritional needs covered. Schedule your mealtimes so that you don't skip meals. Skipping meals won't help you lose weight, if anything; it will only make you hungrier for your next meal. And when your body starts to feel deprived, you'll tend to eat more to make up for the meal you skipped.

Start a routine that will enable you to eat your main meals at the same time every day. You can also include small healthy snacks in the afternoon if you need something to keep your energy levels up, and don't forget to finish your meal with a cup of your favorite detox tea.

Conclusion

Thank you again for downloading this book!

I hope this book was able to help you to get a better insight on how you can use the tea cleanse to get the body and lifestyle that you've always wanted. With the right information and mindset, it's never too late to regain your physical health and improve your quality of life. By understanding fully how a tea detox works and how it can improve your life, you'll be back in shape in no time.

It may not be easy to give up on your old habits altogether, but know that it is possible. As long as you create an action plan that will help you start on the right track, anything is possible.

Make sure to apply what you have learned from this book immediately. You don't have to make drastic change. You just need to do something to jumpstart the process, and doing a healthy tea detox should be enough to help you get that flat tummy you've always wanted.

The 14 Day Paleo Diet Plan

The Paleo Diet For

Beginners Cookbook

Table Of Contents

Introduction

I want to thank you and congratulate you for downloading the book, *"The 14 Day Paleo Diet Plan: The Paleo Diet For Beginners Cookbook"*. This book will teach you all that you need to know about the Paleo Diet, and how it can boost your health.

This book contains proven steps and strategies on how to:

- Make very tasty and healthy meals from scratch

- Enjoy a varied diet that could help you to lose weight and improve your health

- Eat and enjoy food that is highly nutritious, without feeling like you're missing out

- Eat meals that leave you feeling satisfied

- Use the plan long-term if you wish to continue enjoying a healthy, tasty, and balanced diet.

- And so much more!

There's no need for you to put yourself on a very restrictive diet in the hope that you'll become healthy. The Paleo Diet plan will help you to improve your health in no time. Because you will no longer be eating any processed foods, your health will improve, you'll sleep better at night and you'll look better too. It's no wonder more and more people are now enjoying the 14 Day Paleo Diet Plan

Thanks again for downloading this book, I hope you enjoy it!

Chapter 1: The Benefits Of A Paleo Diet Plan

More and more people are now switching to a Paleo diet simply because they have realized how good it is for you. Too many of us eat too many processed foods that aren't doing our bodies any good whatsoever.

A Paleo diet is thought to be similar to the kind of diet cave men and women ate thousands, if not millions of years ago. Their diet was one that consisted of meat (Including fish), fresh fruit and vegetables. They didn't consume dairy products and neither did they consume processed foods, which include cereal products.

Your Body's Preferred Diet

A Paleo diet is simply your bodies preferred diet, as it will contain all of the nutrients that your body needs in order to stay healthy. Our ancestors didn't need to eat processed foods, and neither do we. Although we may have evolved somewhat, and our lives may be far different from our ancestors lives, the nutrients that our bodies need is still very much the same.

Because the Paleo diet is your bodies preferred diet, it means that it's highly sustainable. This means that you can switch to the Paleo diet permanently if you wish, and you won't be doing yourself any harm. Many other diets are not sustainable in the long-term, and they should only be undertaken for a short period of time.

The Paleo diet is different as it offers your body all the nutrients that it needs, and will turn you into a healthy human being that has a lower risk of obesity and diet related illnesses and conditions.

Chapter 2 : Starting The Paleo Diet Plan

If you are undertaking the Paleo diet plan for the very first time, you may appreciate some helpful tips. I know from my own experience that starting a new diet plan can be quite hard. This is why I've decided to include a few tips so that you find your journey a little bit easier.

Making mistakes

We occasionally make mistakes when we embark on a new diet, it happens to all of us. If you accidentally eat something that wouldn't ordinarily be part of the Paleo diet, don't worry, just go back to eating the foods you should eat, as soon as you can. There's nothing you can do about eating something you shouldn't have eaten, just do your best to make sure it doesn't happen again, and put it all down to experience.

Find out where you can source your ingredients

One of the best things you can do before you go ahead and start this diet plan, is to work out where you're going to source your ingredients. If your local stores don't sell much in the way of fresh fruits and vegetables, you will need to work out where you're going to get them from.

Take a trip to your local market, visit a greengrocers nearby, or travel a little further afield to a town that sells the food you're looking for. Some stores may be more than happy to deliver the products you need, right to your door, so why not ask and see if they can help?

Many of the ingredients you'll need in order to make some of the recipes I've included in this book can be made from day to day ingredients. There is nothing fancy that you shouldn't be able to get hold of. Take a look at the food you need, make a list of all the ingredients you want to buy, and get shopping!

Start the plan with a friend

You may be wondering why I have suggested that you start the plan with a friend. I'm suggesting that you do this because it will make the diet a much easier one. Sometimes it's less hassle having someone to compare notes with. What's more is you'll also find that you can motivate each other when things are getting tough. Plus, if you stick to the plan, you can both go out and enjoy rewarding yourself for being good, and that's never a bad thing.

Why not find a friend or even a family member who is willing to take part in the Paleo diet plan with you? If no-one wants to join you, then my suggestion is to look for an online Paleo forum. Forums like these can prove to be very useful as they're bound to be full of hints, tips, recipe ideas, motivation skills and anything else that has kept people going.

Don't do the plan alone, unless you're absolutely confident that you can motivate yourself every day, even when the going gets tough.

Key Foods/Ingredients

Fruits and vegetables

As fresh as possible, try to source them from your local market as they will be extra fresh, they're likely to be a lot cheaper, and you're supporting local businesses too.

If you must eat processed fruit and vegetables, look for those that have very little or no added sugar. Frozen fruit and vegetables is often just as good as fresh, but again, watch out for any added sugar.

Dairy Products

Dairy products should be avoided when you undertake the Paleo plan. This is because most dairy products have been processed, and they're not always very good for you.

Did you know the only milk that our bodies have been made to consume is breast milk? We're not supposed to drink cow's milk as we're unable to digest it properly.

If you would still like to add milk to your diet, I recommend that you consider drinking soy milk, or almond or coconut milk if needs be.

I know it's hard to stay away from dairy products all together, but there are some good and very tasty alternatives. I know these have been processed to a degree, but they ensure that you get the calcium you need, along with other very beneficial nutrients.

Eggs

If you love nothing more than to eat an egg or two, then you will be pleased to know that you can carry on eating them. Eggs are perfectly natural, they haven't been processed, and they are incredibly good for you. Enjoy an egg with your breakfast, or at any other time of the day.

Chapter 3 : Diet Plan (14 Day Guide)

The Paleo diet plan is perhaps one of the healthiest diet plans you're likely to come across. Full of fresh fruits and vegetables, very little or no processed foods, along with meals and snacks that contain very little fat. The great news is that you can enjoy this diet plan, while also consuming a wide variety of foods that you can make from scratch.

Please take a look at the meal plan I have listed below. The plan is merely a suggestion as to what you should eat, you don't have to stick to it. You will find recipes for most of the meals, in the following chapters.

Please note that while a lot of the recipes contain no processed food whatsoever, a few of them do. This is because some of you may find it hard to make the suggested dishes, without using some pre-packaged ingredients.

Remember, there are a lot of dairy alternatives out there, so source and use them when you can.

Day One

Breakfast: Sweet potato waffles

Snack: Apple, banana and ginger muffin

Lunch: Mackerel salad

Snack: A piece of fruit or a yogurt

Dinner: Barbecue chicken

Day Two

Breakfast: Banana and strawberry smoothie

Snack: Apple chips

Lunch: Lentil and garbanzo soup

Snack: A piece of fruit or a yogurt

Dinner: Bean and tomato chili

Day Three

Breakfast: Vegetable tofu scramble

Snack: Coconut, banana and chocolate smoothie

Lunch: Roast chicken wraps

Snack: A piece of fruit or a yogurt

Dinner: Treat yourself to anything you like

Day Four

Breakfast: A piece of fruit, or two

Snack: Fruit salad

Lunch: Chili and celery salad

Snack: A piece of fruit or a yogurt

Dinner: Turkey and nectarine burgers

Day Five

Breakfast: Cherry and quinoa porridge

Snack: Apple, banana and ginger muffin

Lunch: Cilantro and spinach smoothie

Snack: A piece of fruit or a yogurt

Dinner: Steamed salmon and zucchini

Day Six

Breakfast: Orange and lemon smoothie

Snack: Apple chips

Lunch:Pasta and borlotti bean soup

Snack: A piece of fruit or a yogurt

Dinner: Beef Noodles

Day Seven

Breakfast: Trail mix with banana

Snack: Coconut, banana and chocolate smoothie

Lunch: Pear and persimmon salad

Snack: A piece of fruit or a yogurt

Dinner: Baked potato with salad

Day Eight

Breakfast: Sweet potato waffles

Snack: Apple, banana and ginger muffin

Lunch: Mackerel salad

Snack: A piece of fruit or a yogurt

Dinner: Barbecue chicken

Day Nine

Breakfast: Banana and strawberry smoothie

Snack: Apple chips

Lunch: Lentil and garbanzo soup

Snack: A piece of fruit or a yogurt

Dinner: Bean and tomato chili

Day Ten

Breakfast: Vegetable tofu scramble

Snack: Coconut, banana and chocolate smoothie

Lunch: Roast chicken wraps

Snack: A piece of fruit or a yogurt

Dinner: Treat yourself to anything you like

Day Eleven

Breakfast: A piece of fruit, or two

Snack: Fruit salad

Lunch: Chili and celery salad

Snack: A piece of fruit or a yogurt

Dinner: Turkey and nectarine burgers

Day Twelve

Breakfast: Cherry and quinoa porridge

Snack: Apple, banana and ginger muffin

Lunch: Cilantro and spinach smoothie

Snack: A piece of fruit or a yogurt

Dinner: Steamed salmon with zucchini

Day Thirteen

Breakfast: Orange and lemon smoothie

Snack: Apple chips

Lunch: Pasta and borlotti bean soup

Snack: A piece of fruit or a yogurt

Dinner: Beef Noodles

Day Fourteen

Breakfast: Trail mix with banana

Snack: Coconut, banana, and chocolate smoothie

Lunch: Pear and persimmon salad

Snack: A piece of fruit or a yogurt

Dinner: Baked potato with salad

Chapter 4: Paleo Breakfast Recipes

Enjoy a delicious and nutritious breakfast every single morning. If you are a little short on time in the mornings, making your breakfast the night before could help a great deal.

Sweet Potato Waffles

Serves 2

4 tablespoons of cornstarch

4 tablespoons of sweet potato puree

6 tablespoons of wheat pastry flour

Half a teaspoon of salt

4 tablespoons of vegan-friendly buttermilk

2 tablespoons of brown sugar

A quarter of a teaspoon of nutmeg

2 teaspoons of baking powder

2 vegan-friendly eggs

4 tablespoons of vegan-friendly butter (Melted)

118 grams of ham

Method:

Turn on your waffle iron and preheat. Now whisk the cornstarch and add the baking powder, salt, nutmeg, and stir. Take the buttermilk and add it to a different bowl. Add the butter, puree and eggs, and whisk.

Add the flour mixture to the sweet potato mixture, and stir. Add the ham and stir once more. Now spray the waffle iron with some oil and spoon about 80 mls of the mixture into the iron.

Cook until the waffles are golden brown, and serve.

Banana and strawberry smoothie

Serves 1

Ingredients:

1 banana

1 cup of soy or almond milk

A handful of strawberries

1 tablespoon of maple syrup

A pinch of cinnamon

Method:

Add the ingredients to your juicer or blender, and blend until smooth. Pour into a glass and serve.

Orange and lemon smoothie

Serves 1

Ingredients:

A tablespoon of lemon juice

1 orange

Half a grapefruit

1 tablespoon of honey

4 tablespoons of soy based yogurt

240ml of soy milk

Method:

Place the ingredients into your blender or juicer, and blend until smooth. Pour into a glass and serve.

<u>Vegetable Tofu Scramble</u>

Serves 3

Ingredients:

A packet of Tofu (Preferably firm)

3 handfuls of spinach leaves

1 quartered tomato

3 garlic cloves

Half a red onion

Half a bell pepper (Any color)

A pinch of salt

Method:

Take a food processor, and add the spinach, onion, garlic, and pepper. Pulse the ingredients until they are fine. Take a skillet, and add the mixture, cooking on a medium high heat. Once the mixture starts to simmer, add the salt and tofu, and then stir. Cook the ingredients until there's very little liquid left. Serve.

Cherry and Quinoa Porridge

Serves 2

Ingredients:

2 tablespoons of quinoa

240ml water

Half a teaspoon of vanilla extract

1 tablespoon of honey

A quarter of a teaspoon of cinnamon

A handful of unsweetened cherries

Method:

Add all the ingredients apart from the honey, to a pan and place on a medium to high heat. Bring to the boil, and then reduce the heat. Simmer for about 15 minutes, or until the water has dissolved. The quinoa should now be tender. Drizzle with the honey, and serve.

Trail mix

Serves 1

Ingredients:

A handful of sugar-free trail mix

1 banana

Half a glass of soy, almond or coconut milk
(Optional)

Method:

Chop the banana into small pieces and add to
the trail mix, stir to combine.

Add the soy, almond or coconut milk and stir
once more. Serve.

A Piece of fruit, or two

A piece of fruit can be a very healthy breakfast, especially if you don't usually eat at this time of the day. Try to choose a piece of fruit or two that you like, and one that you won't eat again later that day. This is to ensure your body gets as much nutrition as it can from a wide range of fruits.

Chapter 5 : Lunch Time Recipes

These lunch time recipes can be boxed up and taken to work, or enjoyed at home. Eat any leftovers in the next few days so you enjoy them at their freshest.

Mackerel Salad

Serves 2

Ingredients:

3 ounces of un-smoked fresh mackerel

60mls of vegan-friendly mayonnaise

Half a minced clove of garlic

Half a tablespoon of chopped parsley

Half a teaspoon of lemon juice

Half a chopped celery stalk

Half a chopped onion

Method:

Place all of the ingredients apart from the mackerel into a bowl, and stir. Take a fork and separate the mackerel so it flakes. Add the mackerel to the salad, toss to combine and serve.

Roast Chicken Wraps

Serves 3

Ingredients:

3 tablespoons of vegan-friendly mayonnaise

A quarter of a teaspoon of salt

Half a tablespoon of vinegar

Half a teaspoon of black pepper

Half a roasted chicken

2 handfuls of red cabbage, shredded

A pinch of cayenne pepper

1 tablespoon of pickle juice

3 organic whole wheat flat breads

Method:

Place the black pepper, pickle juice, and mayonnaise in a bowl. In another bowl, add the salt, cabbage and cayenne pepper and toss.

Chop the chicken into bite size pieces, and then add to the mayonnaise, and stir. Now spoon out the mayonnaise and cabbage mixtures into the flat breads, roll, and serve.

Chili and Celery Salad

Serves 3

Ingredients:

A sprinkling of chili flakes

4 chopped celery stalks

A tablespoon of lemon juice

1 tablespoon of lemon zest

2 dates (Soaked and pitted)

A tablespoon of tahini

5 grams of chopped parsley

A pinch of salt

10 toasted almonds

Fresh mint to taste

Method:

Put the dates and any liquid they have been soaked in, and place them in a blender. Add the chili, salt, lemon juice and tahini, and blend. When the mixture is smooth, pour the ingredients into a bowl and then add the celery, lemon zest, parsley almonds and salt. Stir and serve.

Pasta and Borlotti Bean Soup

Serves 3

Ingredients:

140 grams of borlotti beans, soaked and drained

Half a medium sized onion, chopped

A clove of minced garlic

Half a celery stalk, sliced

3 chopped tomatoes

Half a tablespoon of olive oil

Half a carrot, sliced

Half a bunch of kale, sliced

125 grams of macaroni

Seasoning

Method:

Add the beans to a large cooking pot, and then fill with water until they are covered by approximately 2 inches. Boil, and then remove any foam from the top. Reduce the heat and then simmer, covered for approximately 40 minutes, or until the beans are nice and tender.

Add the celery, carrot, onion and garlic to another pan and cook until tender (About 8-10 minutes). Drain the beans, and then add them to this pan, along with the tomatoes, salt and about 480 mls of water. Boil, add the pasta and cook until it's reached your preferred consistency. Add the kale and simmer for 5 minutes, and serve.

<u>Lentil and Garbanzo Soup</u>

Serves 4

Ingredients:

1 onion, chopped

1 teaspoon of grated ginger

1 teaspoon of turmeric

A quarter of a teaspoon of cayenne pepper

Half a teaspoon of ground cumin

A handful of chopped carrots

A handful of chopped celery

1 teaspoon of minced garlic

1 can of drained and rinsed Garbanzo beans

2 chopped tomatoes

38 grams of lentils

720ml of vegetable stock

Method:

Sauté the onion in a large pot on a medium to high heat. Now add the celery and carrots, and cook for 5 more minutes. Add the garlic and the remainder of the ingredients, apart from the stock, and cook for 30-40 seconds. Now add the broth and cook for approximately 1 and a half hours, or until the lentils are tender. Serve.

<u>**Cilantro and Spinach Smoothie**</u>

Serves 1

Ingredients:

2 cilantro sprigs

114 grams of spinach

Half a red bell pepper

1 tomato, preferably large, chopped

Half a celery stalk, chopped

A dash of lime juice

Half a carrot, chopped

A quarter of a small onion, chopped

Method:

Add all the ingredients to your juicer or blender, and blend until smooth. Serve.

<u>Pear and Persimmon Salad</u>

Serves 2

Ingredients:

1 persimmon, sliced

1 pear, sliced

1 teaspoon of mustard

3 tablespoons of olive oil

1 minced shallot

2 tablespoons of lemon juice

1 teaspoon of garlic, minced

375 grams of spinach

62 grams of pecan nuts

Method:

Add the mustard, lemon juice, oil, shallot and garlic to a bowl and mix. Now add the persimmon and, pear spinach and pecan nuts and toss. Serve.

Chapter 6 : Dinner Recipes

The following dinner recipes should leave you feeling quite satisfied at the end of the day.

Barbecue Chicken

Serves 2

Ingredients:

1 de-boned chicken breast

2 de-boned chicken thighs

A quarter of a teaspoon of garlic

Three quarters of a tablespoon of paprika

A dash of cayenne pepper

150 grams of barbecue sauce

Method:

Skin the chicken and cut it into thin strips. Add the paprika, garlic, salt and cayenne pepper to a bowl and stir. Now rub the mixture onto the chicken,m and grill for 2 minutes to seal.

Cook the chicken in a pan until it's almost cooked (For about 10 minutes), and then place under the grill once more. Coat the chicken with the barbecue sauce, and cook for an extra minute, and serve.

Bean and Tomato Chili

Serves 3

Ingredients:

1 can of black beans

1 can of chopped tomatoes

Half a can of pinto beans

1 red onion, chopped

1 celery stalk, chopped

Half a bell pepper, chopped

2 cloves of garlic, chopped

1 tablespoon of olive oil

1 tablespoon of cilantro

1 tablespoon of chili powder

1 teaspoon of cumin

Half a teaspoon of oregano

2 pinches of salt

1 teaspoon of lime juice

Three quarters of a teaspoon of paprika

Half a bay leaf

240ml of water

Method:

Using a Dutch oven, pour the olive oil into the bottom and heat. Add the onion, carrot, celery, 1 pinch of salt, and the pepper. Stir. Cook for 5 minutes.

Add the paprika, garlic, chili, oregano, and cumin and stir for 1 minute. Add the pinto beans, black beans, tomatoes, the bay leaf and water, and stir. Bring to a simmer and stir occasionally. Cook for 15 minutes, then add the cilantro and stir once more. Sprinkle in the rest of the salt, stir and serve.

<u>**Turkey and Nectarine Burgers**</u>

Makes: 6-8

500 grams of ground turkey

1 onion, chopped

1 tablespoon of coriander

2 nectarines, chopped

28 grams of sun dried tomatoes, chopped

A handful of cilantro, chopped

2 tablespoons of salt and pepper

Method:

Sauté the onion until it's tender. Place the all of the ingredients into a large bowl and stir thoroughly. Make patties using your hands, shape them into your preferred size, and then place in the refrigerator for a few hours to settle.

Once the burgers have settled, grill them with a touch of oil for about 5 minutes on each side, or until they are cooked. Serve.

Steamed Salmon with Zucchini

Serves 2

Ingredients:

2 salmon fillets

1 small zucchini, sliced

Half a sliced lemon

Half a sliced onion

60ml of water

120ml of white wine

Half a teaspoon of salt

A pinch of ground pepper

Method:

Take a Dutch oven and place the onion, zucchini, lemon, water and white wine in the bottom. Now season the salmon. Place a steamer rack over the ingredients in the Dutch oven. Cook on a medium to high heat until the liquid starts to boil. Reduce the heat, and then place the salmon on the steamer rack and cover. Steam for approximately 8 minutes, or until the salmon is cooked. Serve.

<u>Beef Noodles</u>

Serves 3

Ingredients:

250 grams of ground beef

Half a packet of noodles

Half a green pepper, chopped

2 tomatoes, chopped

1 onion, chopped

100 grams of grated cheese

175 grams of corn

A handful of mushrooms

Salt and pepper to season

Method:

Place the beef in a Dutch oven and cook on a low heat. Cook for 8-10 minutes, or until the beef is cook to your taste. Add the pepper, mushrooms, corn, onions and seasoning, and stir.

Place the noodles on top of the ingredients and sprinkle the grated cheese over the noodles. Take the tomatoes and put them on top of the cheese, and close the lid on the oven. Cook for approximately 1 hour on a medium to high heat. Serve.

Baked Potato with Salad

Serves:1

Ingredients:

1 potato

1 tomato, chopped

A handful of lettuce leaves

A quarter of a cucumber, sliced,

1 tomato, chopped

A dash of olive oil

Seasoning

Method:

Bake the potato in the oven for approximately 1 hour, or until it's cooked. Remove and place to one side. Add the salad to a plate and season. Sprinkle with the olive oil. Place the potato next to the salad, and serve.

Chapter 7: Paelo Diet Snacks

Who says that you cannot enjoy some very tasty snacks as part of the Paleo diet plan? If you're feeling peckish, get stuck in to some of these very tasty snacks.

Apple, Banana and Ginger Muffins

Makes: 12

Ingredients:

200 grams of all-purpose flour

1 tablespoon of baking powder

1 tablespoon of apple cider vinegar

1 teaspoon of ground ginger

1 teaspoon of ground cinnamon

Half a teaspoon of salt

175 grams of apple, sliced

150 grams of sugar

180ml of milk

150 grams of mashed banana

140 grams of crystallized ginger

Method:

Preheat the oven to 400 Fahrenheit, and put a muffin pan to one side. Whisk the flour, sugar, baking powder, salt, ginger and cinnamon and put to one side. In a large bowl, add the milk, banana, apple vinegar and ginger, and stir. Add the flour mixture and stir until the ingredients have just mixed together.

Place in the oven and bake for 15 minutes, or until they are done. Serve and enjoy.

Apple Chips

Serves: 2

Ingredients:

4 apples, sliced

A dash of pumpkin spice

A dash of cinnamon

Method:

Place the apple slices on a cookie sheet, and sprinkle with cinnamon. Place in the oven and cook for 1 hour on 230 Fahrenheit. Turn the apple slices over, and sprinkle cinnamon on the other side, and cook at 200 Fahrenheit for 1 hour.

Now turn the oven off, and keep the apples in there for 1 or 2 hours until they are crisp. Remove the apples from the oven, sprinkle with the pumpkin spice and serve.

Coconut, Banana and Chocolate Smoothie

Serves 1

Ingredients:

1 teaspoon of grated coconut

240ml of coconut water

1 teaspoon of cocoa powder

A handful of spinach

1 banana

Method:

Place all of the ingredients into a juicer or blender, and blend until they have all mixed together. Pour into a glass, serve.

Fruit Salad

Serves: 2

Ingredients:

1 banana

1 apple

4 strawberries

A quarter of a melon, sliced

120ml of fresh orange juice

Method:

Place all of the fruit in a bowl, and mix together. Pour over the fresh orange juice, and stir again. Serve.

<u>Oatmeal and Raisin Cookies</u>

Makes 20

90 grams of oats

300 grams of raisins

125 grams of peanut butter alternative

1 teaspoon of vanilla flavoring

1 teaspoon of baking powder

1 teaspoon of cinnamon

A quarter of a teaspoon of salt

A quarter of a teaspoon of nutmeg

60ml of water

Method:

Set the oven to 350 Fahrenheit, and place 60 grams of the oats in a food processor, and pulse them until they are fine. Add the nutmeg, cinnamon, oat mix, baking powder and salt to a bowl and stir.

Place 150 grams of raisins into the food processor and 60ml of water, and puree. Add the peanut butter and vanilla, and puree. Now add the rest of the raisins, and oats, and add to the oat mix, and stir well.

With a teaspoon, scoop up some of the mixture and place on a cookie sheet. Space the cookies 1 inch apart, and flatten them with the back of your spoon. Cook for approximately 12 minutes or until they cookies have browned. Now transfer them to a cooling rack, allow to cool, and serve.

Chapter 8: Hints and Tips

You may appreciate a few hints and tips to make your journey through the Paleo diet plan a little easier. These tips will help you to lose weight, understand weight loss and advise you as to what you should do if you wish to undertake the plan again.

<u>Water</u>

Water is an absolutely integral part of the Paleo plan and any diet for that matter. Water will not only leave you feeling hydrated, but it can also be used to help speed up weight loss too. This is because it can leave you feeling full, despite this, you should make sure that you don't consume too much water as it can be bad for you. Try to stick to 8 glasses of water a day, and use it to stay hydrated.

Exercise

The 14 day Paleo diet plan won't just help you to eat a better diet, but there's bound to be a bit of weight loss there too. If you plan to exercise while you're undertaking this plan, please make sure that you stick to your regular exercise regime.

You may find it too hard to add extra exercise along with a brand new eating plan. My advice is to only try one new thing at a time. Get used to eating a Paleo diet (If you plan on sticking with it long term), and then add more exercise.

Your Weight Loss

Any weight loss that you achieve as part of this plan is likely to be because you're now consuming less salt, less sugar and less fat. These are usually hidden in processed foods, and because you're consuming less if any at all, then you're likely to lose weight.

When you begin to lose weight, you'll probably lose a lot at first, depending on what you regularly eat. If you stick to this plan long-term, the amount of weight that you lose per week will decrease. This is perfectly normal, and is absolutely nothing to worry about.

If you're not looking to lose weight as part of the Paleo diet plan and you're simply looking to enjoy a healthy diet, then you may still lose a little weight. Not everyone looks to lose weight, some people would prefer to eat a healthy balanced diet first, and consider any weight loss to be secondary.

If You Want To Do The Plan Again

Once you have undertook the Paleo diet plan for 14 days, you will no doubt be feeling and looking better. Chances are you've lost a bit of weight, but you're likely to have more energy and you're probably sleeping better too.

The great thing about the Paleo diet plan is that it's completely sustainable in the long-term. This is because it's a very healthy diet that your body will love, and you won't be missing out on any nutrients.

My advice is to enjoy taking part in the Paleo diet plan, but don't forget to treat yourself from time to time. Treating yourself will make you feel like you've been rewarded, but it will also stop you from getting bored too.

Conclusion

Thank you again for downloading this book!

I hope this book was able to help you to understand how great the Paleo Diet Plan is, and how it can help you improve your health and well-being.

The next step is to source the ingredients you need, and get ready to enjoy some very tasty and highly nutritious meals.

Finally, if you enjoyed this book, then I'd like to ask you for a favor, would you be kind enough to leave a review for this book on Amazon? It'd be greatly appreciated!

Click here to leave a review for this book on Amazon!

Thank you and good luck!